URED DANCER

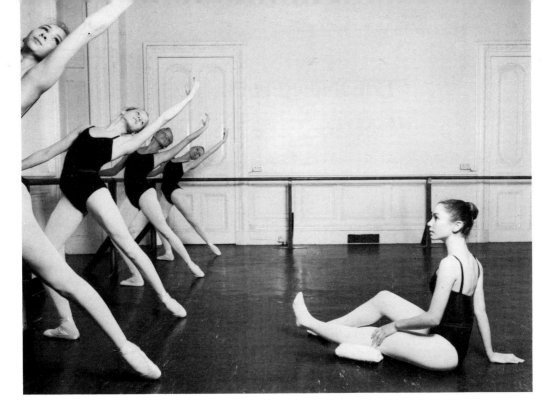

THE
INJURED DANCER

Rachel-Anne Rist
and
Jack Kennedy

Foreword by David Wall
Drawings by Suki Mostyn
Photographs by Michael Bass

WRIGHT

1986 Bristol

Published under the Wright imprint by
IOP Publishing Limited, Techno House, Redcliffe Way,
Bristol BS1 6NX

British Library Cataloguing in Publication Data

Rist, Rachel-Anne
    The injured dancer.
    1. Dancing — Accidents and injuries
    I. Title II. Kennedy, Jack
    617'.1 GV1595

ISBN 0 7236 0894 6

Typeset in Paladium by   Quality Phototypesetting Ltd, Bristol

Printed in Great Britain by   Henry Ling Ltd, Dorset Press, Dorchester

PREFACE

I first became interested in the subject of dance injuries when I had a knee problem that remained undiagnosed through several years of differing opinions, treatments and operations. I was amazed that there was so little real help available to me; indeed, it was suggested to me that I was imagining the whole thing. So I began to try to understand what had gone wrong for myself and soon became fascinated in every aspect of dance injuries. I began to collate all that I found out and related that to the dance class, where injuries often begin. I hope that, through greater understanding of how our bodies work, it may be possible to avoid injury, or at least to recover as quickly and as safely as possible.

I am greatly indebted to Jack Kennedy for his excellent advice and his continued encouragement and support. His help and understanding have been invaluable.

I would also like to thank Mr Jimmy McGregor, Physiotherapist for Manchester United Football Club, for his helpful and constructive opinions. Thanks also to Mr Don Gatherar, Honorary Physiotherapist to the British Olympic Association and British Amateur Athletic Board, for his advice.

Finally, thanks to Mrs M. I. Jack, and Miss Cara Drower and other staff and students of the Arts Education School, Tring; and to my family for their love and support.

ABOUT THE AUTHORS

Rachel-Anne Rist is a ballet teacher at the Arts Educational School, Tring. She has also spent several years teaching dance abroad — in Italy, Canada and the U.S.A. — with experience in teaching from beginners' to professional level. In addition, she has taught an anatomy course for teachers.

Jack Kennedy is a chartered physiotherapist working in Manchester, who has had considerable experience in treating injuries to dancers of all types. He has worked closely with visiting dance companies in Manchester.

CONTENTS

ILLUSTRATIONS

FOREWORD

A dancer's quest for technical perfection in an art form undoubtedly the most physically demanding of all inevitably puts both student and professional at a high risk of injury.

The occurrence of this risk factor makes not only for pain and discomfort but for depression, frustration and impatience. With a prior awareness of the causes, symptoms and treatment of the common dance injury this physical and mental ordeal can be alleviated and, in turn, enhance recovery.

With ever greater demands being made on the dancer's body, this book by Rachel-Anne Rist and Jack Kennedy, who on many occasions advised and treated me during my dancing career, is most welcome and their expertise will assist the search for physical and technical perfection in the dancer.

David Wall

INTRODUCTION

As the standard of ballet technique becomes higher, so more demands are placed upon the dancer and the teacher. As the competition continues to grow, so a dancer is pushed further to the physical limits. The idea of a 'perfect dancer's body' is possibly an enigma. Most students studying dancing do not have a perfect physique and so, as they seek to perform a perfect art with an imperfect instrument, the result will be injuries.

To some extent, a dancer leads most of life in pain. But he or she must also listen carefully to the body when pain is beyond that which is normal and becomes a career-threatening injury. At the back of every dancer's mind must be the question: 'Is this the injury that will stop me dancing?'.

Unfortunately, a dancer's special physiological and psychological needs do not seem to be well met by the medical profession. Therefore, it is the responsibility of every dancer and teacher to understand fully the anatomical structures they work with every day; to assess accurately possible damage and to know what to do about it. Once an injury has occurred, it is vital to receive prompt and correct treatment and make a carefully planned return to full recovery. But, most importantly, the dancer and teacher must find out why the injury occurred and what must be done to prevent future problems.

This book is in no way intended to replace medical advice. Professional help should always be sought at the earliest opportunity. It is intended that students should help themselves to recover more quickly with a full understanding of their injury and so help their doctors or physiotherapists.

INJURIES

Dancers' injuries can fall into two categories — 'over-use' injuries and traumatic injuries.

1. OVER-USE INJURIES
Most injuries fall into this category. They can be caused by a variety of reasons, *all* of which can be prevented.

(a) **Poor technique** A dancer has not corrected the alignment of the body and puts severe and re-occurring strain on a weak set of muscles.

(b) **Repetition** Constant, unnecessary repetition will cause fatigue and will not improve on exercise. Sensitive teaching is required to allow a group of hard-working muscles to relax.

(c) **Structural variation** A growing dancer failing to make body adjustments and re-aligning the centre of weight.

(d) **Muscular imbalance** An over-developed set of muscles will usually leave an underdeveloped set of opposing muscles. For example, the strong muscles at the back of the calf are more developed than those on the front of the leg.

(e) **Equipment** Dancing on a floor that is too hard and does not 'give' will cause many injuries, such as 'shin splints' and stress fractures. Shoes that are too soft and fail to give support to the foot will lead to ankle problems. Ribbons incorrectly tied or tied too tightly will restrict the Achilles tendon. The wearing of good, sensible footwear away from class and performance is equally important in preventing injury.

(f) **Postural defects** Repeated bad habits and an awkward physique are possibly the most common sources of most sports and dance injuries.

2. TRAUMATIC INJURIES

A traumatic injury is caused by a sudden and unexpected accident. It may take the form of a fracture, tear or rupture. Frequently seen traumatic injuries include: broken foot or ankle, strains or tears of the groin or hamstring muscles, dislocation of knee-cap, fracture of tibia and strained back muscles. All these injuries should receive immediate medical attention.

WHAT TO LOOK FOR

When dealing with over-use injuries, there are various signs to look for which can give an indication of the severity of the problems.

Look for signs of a change in skin temperature and colour. The injured site may be very hot and deep pink or purple, or it may be quite cold and pale. Heat at the site of an injury could indicate that the body's own defence mechanism is working. Cold skin temperature could indicate very poor circulation, probably because the injured part has been kept immobile.

Any sign of swelling means that there is something wrong. Suspect the worst and ice-pack as soon as possible. Swelling could be caused by bleeding, or from tissue fluids seeping into the surrounding soft tissues, which is called oedema.

Check for muscle tone above and below the injury. A dancer's muscle balance can alter drastically and very quickly if an injury is present. Wasting (atrophy) must be corrected as soon as possible, as it can lead to further problems.

Do not be over-cautious in feeling for the exact site of pain. Use firm pressure to elicit a response, checking the opposite limb in case of hyper-sensitivity and as a point of reference. Do not be misled and keep rechecking for the exact site of pain.

In making compensatory movements to avoid an over-use injury, a dancer can unconsciously make adjustments and so stress the body in a different place. In trying to avoid the primary site of pain, adjustments made will cause pain in a secondary place. Always find out exactly what movements cause pain and if weight-bearing will heighten the sensation.

REHABILITATION AND SELECTIVE REST

If an injury is totally ignored, further physical damage will be done. If the dancer stops dancing completely, psychological damage will be done and probably stiffness and wasting will occur. The dancer should aim at reaching a happy balance between these two choices: 'selective rest'. This means that, without disregarding medical opinion, the dancer is the best person to judge how much to work and how much to rest. As long as the injury is not stressed by exercise, the dancer can then work to keep the rest of the body in training, yet at the same time be sufficiently aware of the injury to avoid anything that hurts. The aim is to select carefully how much work will keep the body fit, whilst resting the injury.

The cause of the pain must be found and eliminated as far as possible. Strapping or padding is useful to support and protect the injury. This may also help to remind the dancer not to use the injured part. All painful movements should be avoided both during and after selective rest. Some injuries, however, respond well to gentle passive movements to improve mobility and increase circulation. The injury should be well protected during dancing and walking. It is often forgotten by both dancer and teacher to examine how activities outside the studio can affect the injury. Correct walking shoes are important and can add speed to recovery.

Rehabilitation should begin with some gentle stretching, strengthening and non-weight-bearing exercises on the floor. Exercises should be designed to strengthen the muscles surrounding the injury, as wasting can occur very quickly. It is important not to overtire weakened muscles and it is better to do a little and often rather than a lot all at once.

Physical therapy will help keep full range of movement without stressing the injury. Massage will help rid muscles of any fibrous adhesions that may have formed and will stimulate circulation.

If the dancer is exercising on the floor and not weight bearing, there is no chance of aggravating the injured spot. This recovery time should be seen as a chance to re-evaluate strengths and weaknesses. It should be a time to work hard on basic postures and placing. It is also an opportunity for the teacher and dancer to try to understand why the injury occurred and what must be done to prevent it from happening again.

After doing floor exercises for sufficient time, the dancer could progress to participating in some class work. All extensions should be kept low, minimum turn-out used and very little repetition made. The dancer must be careful at this point not to get carried away with pleasure to be back dancing and so forget to limit performance!

Jumps and pointe work should not be done for quite a long time, as they will stress a weakened area. While the rest of the class continues, the injured dancer should then wrap up warmly and do some strengthening exercises on the floor to work the warm muscle gently.

If a dancer has been injured for a week, it will often be at least double that time before full class work should be attempted, and a further week before recovery is complete. It is important that this rather slow process is not rushed and so open the way for further injury. If there is as much as 10 per cent difference in strength and movement between the injured part and the rest of the body, then recovery is incomplete.

It is important to mention that although most conditions affecting a dancer's life will be mechanical, technical and physical, symptoms that appear to relate to bones, joints and muscles can also relate to some other underlying organic problem in the body.

It cannot be stressed too much that a dancer should seek medical advice at an early stage for an accurate assessment to be made. For example, an aching in the joints that one might think was an over-use injury could, in fact, be a virus-related illness that requires a very different approach.

If the physical signs and symptoms are combined with a general feeling of illness, fever or debility and loss of weight, then a more complicated medical problem would be suspected. So, always be on guard for other seemingly non-related symptoms and be prepared to seek help as soon as possible.

It is worth noting also that occasionally the emotional state of the student or dancer can aggravate the problem. Whilst having an injury can be a very traumatic time, it does not help recovery if the patient is rather hysterical. A calm and intelligent approach should be arrived at once initial shock or upset has been overcome.

ANKLES AND FEET

Ankles and feet are subject to an enormous amount of stress. Female dancers, especially, have problems because they have to go en pointe. The ankles often have to deal with five to eight times the body's weight which is transmitted through the feet and legs when landing from jumps.

The most important group of muscles related to the use of the feet are the calf muscles: the gastrocnemii and the soleus. The gastrocnemii are rather large, fleshy, superficial muscles which flex the knee and ankle. The soleus is a deep muscle which flexes only the ankle. These two muscles unite to form the strong Achilles tendon at the back of the ankle.

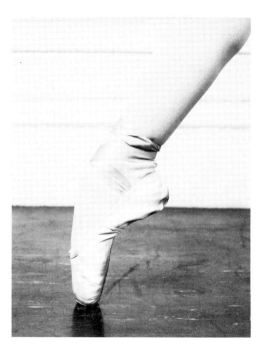

The foot.

The Achilles tendon is non-elastic and is very rarely stretched. Thus, if a dancer suffers a severe rupture of the tendon, it is unlikely that recovery will be sufficient to perform properly again. Students with rather short Achilles tendons and, therefore, small demi-pliés , will find jumps a problem. They often tend to develop very strong feet in compensation for the lack of pliés and this should be encouraged as much as possible. Stretching the calf well before class can help, but very little can be done actually to lengthen the tendon.

It is vital that medical attention be sought at the earliest opportunity should an injury develop in this muscle group or tendon.

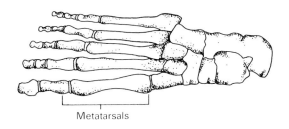

Metatarsals

SPRAINED ANKLE

This is a traumatic injury with severe pain of the ankle — usually on the outside of the foot.

CAUSES

Landing badly from a jump, so that the foot sickles inwards, often tearing ligaments on the outside of the foot.

Falling 'off' a shoe, falling down a stair, or simply tripping up over an object and putting the weight on the outside of the foot can have the same effect.

SYMPTOMS

Pain on the lateral side of the foot, especially when the foot is moved inwards.

Weight-bearing of any kind is usually too painful.

Bruising and swelling often occur quite quickly. There is possibly swelling on the inside of the ankle also, as the medial ligament may be crushed if the lateral ligament is overstretched.

TREATMENT

Medical help must be sought as soon as possible. Ice-packs will help reduce any swelling and so allow the foot to be examined more closely.

If the sprain is severe, medical opinion may suggest that the ruptured ligaments be rested and a walking plaster cast be left on for a couple of weeks.

Careful strapping of the foot to give support.

Physiotherapy, once healing has begun, will help stimulate recovery, which can take between three to six weeks and, in severe cases, six to nine months.

CORRECTION

Exercises to strengthen the foot, ankle and calf muscles. A 'wobble' board is a good way to build up strength.

Other exercises include: circling the foot as much as possible whilst keeping the leg still, sit with calf resting upon knee of other leg and draw circles with the foot outwards and inwards.

Isometric exercises (pushing against pressure) will also help strengthen ankles. Start with the foot sickled inwards and push outwards, against pressure, away from the body. Repeat the opposite way, pushing the foot inwards. These exercises will help strengthen the outside of the calf muscles.

This injury is more common in dancers with sway-back legs and a predisposition to weak legs and feet.

Teachers should watch carefully to make sure that the ankle is well supported in pliés and jumps and that the weight of the body is properly held over the centre of the foot.

TENDONS OF THE ANKLE

The tendons on the inside and outside of the foot are responsible for supporting the foot, and it is important that they are equally strong — an imbalance in strengths gives a predisposition to injury. Two of the most important tendons in the foot are the tibialis anterior and the tibialis posterior. These tendons come from muscles that originate in the calf.

CAUSES

Pain on either the inside or outside of the foot can be caused by incorrect technique. Sickling the foot inwards or outwards over a long period of time will weaken the tendons and could cause strain. Incorrect placement of weight either when walking or dancing may also result in tendon pain.

SYMPTOMS

A general aching in the area with possible swelling or local heat. Jumping will cause pain and so will pointe work or rises.

TREATMENT

Supportive taping will help the dancer to do some movement. Ice-packing, followed by physiotherapy and rest from all painful movements.

CORRECTION

Ankle circling exercises to work the foot and calf muscles. 'Wobble board' work to encourage greater strength and stability. Technique must be closely examined to check for correct weight placement and to avoid sickling the foot.

FRACTURE OF THE FIFTH METATARSAL

This causes pain on the outside of the foot. It may be either a traumatic or an over-use injury.

CAUSES

A sudden fracture may be caused by a direct blow on the foot bones, landing badly from a jump or even by falling off pointe.

An over-use fracture could result from the pull of muscles which can stress the bone and actually bend it. One of the outside calf muscles (peroneus brevis) which orginates on the fibula and inserts into the long fifth metatarsal bone, will begin to pull on the foot bone if used incorrectly.

SYMPTOMS

Pain on the outside of the foot during all weight-bearing activities.

Some swelling may be present.

Squeezing the foot bones laterally would also elicit pain.

This fracture would probably appear on an X-ray. In cases of a traumatic fracture, the dancer may even hear the bone break.

TREATMENT

Most weight-bearing activities should be kept to a minimum. Doctors may suggest a plaster cast to ensure recovery, supportive taping and, as healing progresses, institute faradic foot baths and intensive foot exercises.

If the foot does not need immobilization, wearing clogs could help to avoid pressure on the bone when walking. Recovery may extend over a period of six weeks.

CORRECTION

Isometric exercises, as previously described, to work the calf muscles. Foot circling and flexing.

'Wobble board' work and slow rises with the foot firstly parallel and then turned out.

If there is a tendency towards instability in the ankle, strengthening exercises should be done to prevent the likelihood of this injury. Exercises should be repeated many times at any one time to gain real strength. One hundred times repeated twice to six times daily will make a real difference to ankle strength.

STRESS FRACTURE OF METATARSALS AND DROPPED METATARSAL HEAD

With these injuries pain is experienced underneath the 'knuckle' of the toe joint — they may be related to any of the toes.

CAUSES

Both these injuries are over-use injuries and may result from similar causes. These include: an increase in work load or a change in technique, and incorrect dance technique with body weight poorly aligned. May possibly be caused by dancing bare foot or by extra pressure put upon the ball of the foot. Very high heels worn outside dancing would irritate the problem.

SYMPTOMS

Pain underneath the foot in 'pushing off' in jumps, or when on the demi-pointe. Walking also causes pain. The fracture of the metatarsal may be known as a 'march' fracture as it often occurs because of frequent walking on hard surfaces.

TREATMENT

In the case of dropped metatarsal head, carefully applied strapping, with support directly underneath the bone, should allow the dancer to continue some activity. All painful movements should be avoided. A stress fracture of the metatarsals should be treated medically. A plaster cast is not usually necessary. Recovery time is about 6 weeks.

CORRECTION

Once symptom free, exercises should be done to strengthen the muscles underneath the foot. Lifting the metatarsal arch up, whilst keeping the toes on the floor, will work the small foot muscles. Electrical stimulation, as advised by a chartered physiotherapist, will help encourage the muscles to support the foot properly. Check dance technique to ensure correct weight placement.

SESAMOID BONE FRACTURE

This is an over-use injury due to repeated direct pressure on the ball of the foot.

CAUSES

The two sesamoid bones in the foot are found underneath the joint of the first toe and first metatarsal head. As these bones are not visible and cannot normally be felt, a dancer is usually unaware of their existence. However, constant use of the foot on a hard surface will greatly irritate the bones, and the bursa betweeen them. Tap dancers tend to suffer more than any other dancer, because the weight of the body is carried well forwards on the balls of the feet, and the area is subject to repeated stress.

SYMPTOMS

Soreness and aching underneath the ball of the foot. Pain when on a rise on the half toe.

Walking may also produce pain as the bones take the weight of the body in the propulsion forward. The fracture should be visible in an X-ray.

TREATMENT

If the fracture is complete, a surgeon may recommend an operation to remove the broken bone. The incision is usually at the

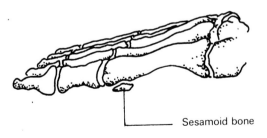

Sesamoid bone

side of the joint and not directly underneath the foot. This way any resulting scar tissue will not interfere with weight bearing in the future. Initial treatment would attempt to reduce the inflammation by rest, padding support to redistribute pressure away from the bones concerned. A felt pad underneath the ball of the foot, with a piece cut out where the sore sesamoid bone is located, will relieve it of weight bearing and so lessen the pressure placed on it.

Chiropodist's felt

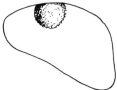

Cut away excess and shape round ball of foot

CORRECTION

Little can be done to correct or prevent this injury. Rises and jumps should be kept to a minimum, or avoided until the inflammation has subsided. Often, several weeks' recovery time is required. Many dancers, when X-rayed years later for a separate injury, reveal their fractures although they have caused no problems.

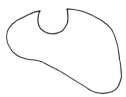

Place under foot with cut-out directly under sore area

Sesamoid bone pad to relieve pressure.

DROPPED ARCH

This is an over-use injury resulting in an ache underneath the foot.

CAUSES

Incorrect technique which allows the ankles to roll inwards and so place excessive weight on the inside of the foot. If turn-out is not properly sustained in the hips, and the whole leg is allowed to rotate inwards, whilst forcing the foot outwards, the longitudinal ligaments in the foot may become weak from incorrect placement of the weight.

This injury often occurs in conjunction with a bunion, or knee problems related to poor turn-out.

SYMPTOMS

Tenderness in the long muscles which run underneath the big toe joint to the heel on the inside of the foot.

Aching after exercise, or even just walking. There may be stiffness in the big toe joint because the ligaments that go under the foot and end in the big toe become inelastic and so sensitive to stretching.

TREATMENT

Physiotherapy will help by either ultrasound therapy or by electrical stimulation (faradic) to encourage better use of the muscles and so strengthen them.

During recovery, a small arch support will ease the aching by taking the weight off the area and will encourage the dancer to put more weight on the outside of the foot, so distributing the weight more effectively.

CORRECTION

Exercises to stimulate the small muscles of the foot.

Keeping the foot flat on the floor and the toes still, try to lift up the arch and hold before releasing. Maintain this lift, rising smoothly on to three quarter foot, and then slowly sink through the foot.

Try picking up a pen with the toes and holding it. Sit with the legs straight and the feet flexed upwards, contract and clench the feet tightly together and hold before relaxing. This should be done alternately with trying to spread the toes evenly sideways.

Check technique to ensure the foot is properly supported during exercise, the weight is evenly distributed (especially in plié) and that the turn-out is properly maintained.

HALLUX VALGUS (BUNION)

This causes inflammation, tenderness and/or enlargement of the big toe joint. It is an over-use injury.

CAUSES

This is caused by rolling the foot and ankle forwards. Too much weight is then taken on to the big toe joint, and not evenly distributed throughout the foot. Causes may also be related to not sustaining the turn-out and poor technique. Very close, tight-fitting shoes will aggravate the problem.

SYMPTOMS

The joint of the big toe may become enlarged or inflamed. The big toe itself is often forced laterally towards the other toes.

Pain will be felt on weight-bearing with the ankle rolling inwards. Sometimes, even walking can be painful.

The bursa (cushion) that protects the delicate toe joint becomes reddened and inflamed.

Dance shoes become worn and marked where the bunion is.

TREATMENT

Severe cases need medical advice and perhaps surgery. A pad could be worn over the joint to stop direct pressure on the bursa. Weight should be taken off the joint by ensuring that the ankles are not rolling forwards. The big toe must be brought back in line with the joint. This can be done by placing a small pad of either sponge or chiropodist's felt between the first two toes, and then strapping it into position with 1 inch tape. Physiotherapy may include ice-packing and ultrasound, with mobilization of the joint and foot exercises.

CORRECTION

The first thing to do is to check technique. If turn-out is limited from the hip socket, compensation may be made in the knee and translated into over-turning out the feet. The weight of the body then falls incorrectly. The weight must be firmly held on the three points of balance: the heel, fifth metatarsal and first metatarsal head.

Tight-fitting shoes must be avoided and soft dance shoes, not pointe shoes, should be worn.

It may be helpful to use an arch support insole inserted into regular shoes to encourage weight to shift to the outside of the foot, and so ease the pressure off the joint.

With some slight degree of hallux valgus, exercises can be done to strengthen the weak muscles of the toe. A good way to do this is to loop a piece of strong, thick, elastic around the big toe, and hold the ends. By pushing down gently against the elastic and slowly releasing, relaxing and repeating, the toe muscles (flexor hallus brevis and longus) will be encouraged to strengthen.

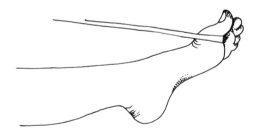

Exercise to strengthen the big toe muscles.

HALLUX RIGIDUS

This is stiffness in the big toe joint.

CAUSES

May be caused by inelasticity of the muscles that go into the big toe underneath the foot. Possible incorrect placement of weight on the big toe joint when on demi-pointe.

SYMPTOMS

Very little range of movement in the joint. The big toe is usually incapable of much upwards movement. Pain on demi-pointe, local tenderness and possibly swelling. Inability to 'push off' the foot in jumps.

TREATMENT

Because of the great importance of this joint to the dancer, it is hard to decide how best to treat this condition. Unless pain is very severe, the dancer may be able to continue activity to some extent.

CORRECTION

Work to maintain as much mobility as possible in the joint whilst avoiding painful movements. Check that weight placement is correct when on demi-pointe and full pointe. If it is decided that the condition needs surgery, it should be emphasized that this option should be chosen at the end of a dancing career.

ACHILLES TENDONITIS

Pain is felt at the back of the heel by the Achilles tendon, approximately 2 inches above the top of the heel bone. This is generally an over-use injury.

CAUSES

Choreography which is too rapid and does not allow the heels time to get down on the floor.

Dancing on a very hard floor that does not 'give'.

Very short tendons being subjected to a lot of jumps with inadequate warm-up.

Trying to force a foot 'over' too far in pointe shoes.

SYMPTOMS

Pain on knee bends, jumps and even pointing the foot.

There may be some fluid build-up in response to inflammation.

In rare cases, some fibrous nodules (or bumps) may appear around the tendon.

The ankle is usually very stiff to walk on first thing in the morning.

TREATMENT

Complete rest from jumps and pointe work.

Heel lifts inserted into dance shoes and regular shoes will allow the tendon to relax more.

Physiotherapy may include ice and ultrasound, combined with firm supportive taping and massage to the calf.

CORRECTION

Non-weight bearing exercises to stretch gently

calf muscles and tendon. It is important to keep as much elasticity in the tendon as possible.

Exercises to stretch calf muscles: sit with leg straight and foot flexed; then, by reaching forwards and cupping the foot with the hands, gently pull the foot towards the body and so stretch the calf muscles where they form the Achilles tendon.

If this is too painful, another way to stretch the calf muscles is to lie face downwards and lift the leg, bent at the knee, with the foot flexed. Allow someone to exert gentle downwards pressure on the foot to stretch the tendon and calf muscles. A stronger exercise may be done at a later stage.

Standing a short distance away from a wall, lean on the wall with the hands flat, back straight and knees straight. Press the heels firmly down onto the floor. Press up to the wall trying to keep the heels down and the back straight.

Make sure the dancer always stretches the muscle group well, prior to class.

Shoes with ribbons should be avoided in recovery. It is vital to stress that ribbons should never be tied at the back of the calf, but on the inside of the ankle where the knot will not inhibit tendon movement.

A slow return to class work and, finally, jumps, once recovery is made. Emphasis should be placed on getting the heels firmly down on the floor in pliés and all landings from jumps.

If treated correctly, recovery may only take a few weeks. Treated incorrectly, it may be many months. Difficult cases require expert orthopaedic advice.

BURSITIS OF THE ACHILLES TENDON

This causes pain at the back of the heel by the tendon.

CAUSES

Too much direct pressure on the heel — possibly tight-fitting shoes rubbing against the heel. The cushion, or bursa, behind the tendon becomes inflamed.

Too much forced pointe work because of stiffness in ankle joints developing over several weeks.

Pain at this site can also be caused by a small accessory bone that is present in some dancers.

SYMPTOMS

Soreness and tenderness around the heel, sometimes localized on either side of the tendon.

Pain on jumps, pliés and stretching the foot.

Pinching the area beneath the tendon is painful and usually there is swelling. However, the tendon itself is not necessarily sore.

Sometimes a small lump can be detected.

TREATMENT

Rest from activity which produces soreness.

Physiotherapy may include ice-packing to reduce inflammation and ultrasound to stimulate recovery.

If the case is severe, an orthopaedic surgeon may consider surgery to remove the bursa.

Supportive taping with firm pressure when resting can help considerably.

CORRECTION

Make sure shoes are not too stiff and that draw-strings are not pulled up too tightly in ballet shoes.

Soften the backs of tap or character shoes, or insert cushion into the heel.

As much gentle calf-stretching as possible to maintain elasticity in the tendon.

'DANCER'S HEEL'

This results in pain at the back of the heel with restricted flexion in the foot.

CAUSES

Dancing on a floor that is too hard.

Excessive pointe work which overloads the heel.

A change in dance technique or style, or a change of teacher.

SYMPTOMS

Pain on demi-pointe — not necessarily on full pointe.

Difficulties in jumping and knee bends.

Inability to flex the foot as fully as the opposite limb.

TREATMENT

Good massage to the calf and mobilization of the heel. It eases within days if caught early enough.

CORRECTION

Check movements daily to control the amount of stiffness present and be careful not to force the foot over in pointe shoes.

POINTE WORK

A fairly obvious comment about pointe work is that it is vital that the shoes are correct for the foot. If necessary, high vamps to protect over-arched feet must be used. Another helpful hint for girls with a high arch is to place a wide tube of elastic over the shoe and over the metatarsal arch. This should be between 4 and 5 inches wide and will give the foot extra support until the ankle is stronger.

Ribbons may also be lined with strong seam binding to give added support to the ankle.

Pointe work should never begin until the girl is over the age of 12 years when the bones of the foot have ossified sufficiently to take the weight of the body.

It is interesting to note that the metatarsals will also thicken in response to pointe work and the extra demands made upon the foot. Once pointe work has permanently ceased, then the 5 metatarsal bones will reduce back to their original size. This may help to explain why dancers' feet become slightly wider when they go into full-time classes with a great deal of pointe work.

SHINS AND CALVES: 'SHIN SPLINTS'

'Shin splints' is a phrase used to describe pain in the leg. It is not a true medical condition, but a term dancers use to describe pain in that context. It is a very common injury in dancers. The majority of shin splint pain is related to the front of the leg by the tibia. Some dancers, however, have pain on the outside of the calf by the fibula.

CAUSES

Quite often, the pain is caused by dancing on a very hard floor which does not give. It can also be caused by a change in technique or a change in teachers, an increase in activity and, especially, an increase in jumps. Dancers with weak feet or sway-back legs will often have a tendency to suffer from shin splint pain caused by a microscopic tearing of the muscles of the bone which, in turn, causes a hardening of the lining of the muscle. Blood will then seep into tissue and cause aching and inflammation.

The problem can also be caused by a muscular imbalance. The muscles on the front of the shin (dorsi flexors) tend to be rather weak, as a dancer is nearly always using the muscles at the back of the calf (plantar flexors) to stretch the foot. This imbalance in muscle strengths will mean that one set of muscles works harder than another set and this can lead to injury.

Not getting the heels firmly down on the floor in jumps will also encourage shin splint pain.

SYMPTOMS

Pain down the inside of the tibia (main

weight-bearing bone) or on the outside of the calf by the fibula during hard exercise, especially jumps. There may be some local tenderness around the area and possibly some swelling.

TREATMENT

Very little can be done to ease the aching. An ice-pack on the bone and surrounding area will discourage inflammation and give relief from symptoms. The leg should then be elevated and allowed to rest.

Jumps and pointe work should be avoided. A doctor may prescribe anti-inflammatory tablets or recommend physiotherapy in the form of ultrasound which will aid recovery.

Sometimes, gentle massage of the inflamed area will stimulate circulation and so aid recovery — this should be a very gentle, not deep, massage. Supportive strapping should be applied at the earliest opportunity by the physiotherapist.

CORRECTION

Exercises to strengthen all lower leg muscles should be done.

Work on the 'wobble' board which will stimulate all ankle, calf and thigh muscles.

Ankle circling, keeping the calf still and moving the foot inwards and outwards, with frequent repetitions, will slowly strengthen the muscles.

Isometric exercises (pushing against pressure) to work the weak front of the shin muscles. Sit with the leg straight out in front, foot stretched and then pull the foot upwards, as if to flex the foot against steady pressure. Do this the opposite way, pushing the foot slowly downwards and also do this for the toes, keeping the foot stretched, working the toes upwards and downwards.

All these exercises must be done little and often. Overworking a set of tired muscles will produce cramp, not strength. Work the muscles until just before they begin to tire and then stop, rest and relax before repeating.

The dancer can continue with as much class as possible, as long as there is no pain. Once jumps begin, the dancer should sit down and begin to go through the calf exercises.

Shin splint problems related to the fibula will be aggravated by rises onto the half toe so, again, these should be avoided.

As the dancer slowly returns to join in full class with jumps, there should be plenty of time to rest and stretch calf muscles between exercises.

Aerobic dancers tend to suffer from shin problems because of the amount of jumps on two legs or one leg with no time to rest. If all previously described exercises do not help, try wearing either a training shoe or a tennis

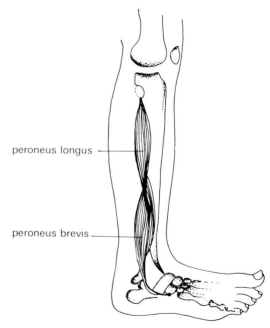

Peroneal calf muscles.

pump with a slightly raised heel, as this will help put the body weight into the heels and less on the front of the shin.

A sensitive teacher can sometimes spot a likely candidate for shin splint problems. The dancer will have some degree of sway-back legs, weak feet and ankles and a poor sense of 'bounce' in elevation. Preventative measures should be taken to encourage better use of the legs.

STRESS FRACTURE OF TIBIA AND FIBULA

A stress fracture is an over-use injury; the most common is of the tibia at the front of the shin. The fibula, at the lateral side of the leg, is a non-weight bearing bone and is not exposed to the same pressures. However, the fibula can have a stress fracture caused by the strong pull of the peroneal calf muscles off the insertion into the bone.

Stress fractures of the tibia and fibula will have a long history of shin splint pain.

CAUSES

The fracture is caused by repeated pressure, or fatigue, in a bone, which causes the bone to 'bend'. After repeated over-use, a small slit appears in the bone.

Stress fractures happen more often in women than in men because women have a less compact skeleton.

Insufficent rest and recovery time during the initial few weeks of shin splint pain will cause the already weakened bone to fracture.

SYMPTOMS

After a few months of repeated over-use and pain, a hard lump can be felt on the bone.

There is pain on all weight-bearing movements, even walking.

Aching and tenderness around the area.

The stress fracture of the fibula will cause pain and some discomfort in the outside calf muscle and, when on a rise, tenderness will also be felt about 2 inches above the ankle bone.

It is possible to have multiple stress

fractures on the same bone if the dancer has continued to work with pain for a long time. An X-ray can help confirm diagnosis, but judgement is far more important.

TREATMENT

Medical advice should be sought.

Treatment must be complete rest from dancing and from all unnecessary weight-bearing activity for several weeks, depending upon the doctor's opinion.

Sometimes it is decided to apply a plaster cast to aid recovery.

If the fracture of the weight-bearing tibia is severe, some form of surgery may be recommended, although this is a rare occurrence.

CORRECTION

As recovery time for this injury can vary between a few weeks and a few months, it is important to keep in training. Floor exercises which are non-weight-bearing and will not aggravate the stress fracture will maintain technique and strength.

When the dancer is advised to return slowly to dancing, great care must be taken to keep most exercises on two legs and avoid sudden movements or jumps. Correct muscular balance in the calf must be restored as soon as possible. (*See* exercises for shin splints p. 30.)

KNEES

Knees are normally very robust and are
bound by strong ligaments and tendons.
Knees are then supported by strong muscles
above, below and behind. They are subject to
enormous pressures in dancing, as they act as
shock-absorbers and as a springing
mechanism to propel the dancer upwards.
Any restrictions in the hip socket, or lack of
ankle strength, will often result in a knee
injury.

The femur (which is the longest bone in
the body) rests upon the main lower leg bone,
the tibia. The patella is a small bone which is
placed in front of the joint of the femur and
the tibia and serves to protect as well as acting
as an attachment for strong thigh muscles.

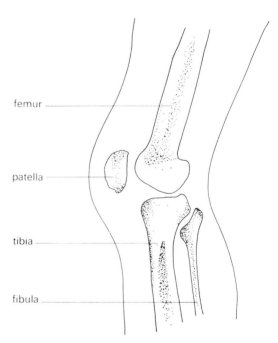

The knee joint.

The quadriceps femoris is a name given to a group of four muscles on the front of the thigh. They unite to form a tendon into which the patella is set. This group of muscles is responsible for lifting the leg and extending the knee upon the thigh.

If a knee has an injury, the quadriceps will tend to atrophy (waste) rather rapidly. This will then cause an imbalance in the muscle tone, which will further encourage injury. Normally, the relative strengths of the quadriceps and femoris and the biceps femoris (or hamstrings, at the back of the thigh) will be approximately 60 per cent and 40 per cent. It is important that this ratio is maintained to avoid further stress injuries. In most knee injuries, the hamstrings tend to shorten if not regularly stretched whilst doing quadriceps exercises. This can lead to further problems around the knee, so a good stretching of the hamstring should complement all quadriceps exercises.

If the muscles above and below the knee are not equally balanced, the patella may be pulled off-centre and be predisposed to dislocate laterally. It is important that all ligaments pull equally to hold the patella firmly in place.

A certain degree of 'bow-legs' is normal amongst dancers. They tend to have well-developed muscles in the legs which can therefore make the legs appear slightly bent in an arabesque. Usually, these legs are good for all steps of elevation.

Another common problem can be 'sway-back' legs. This is when muscles and ligaments are rather long and the leg appears to sway-back at the knees. Aesthetically, these legs are most appealing to look at, as they are often combined with a well arched foot. Adage, and (for girls) pointe work, will be the strongest sections for this kind of leg, and it will be weak for jumps. This is often because the quadriceps are not well used and rarely strong enough. Any mild degree of either bow-legs or sway-back legs, or ideally a combination of the two, is trainable. More care must be given to sway-back legs as they can often lead to future problems due to lack of strength. However, a pronounced exaggeration of either shape of leg will rarely be able to cope fully with the demands made upon it.

Once a knee is damaged, it tends to be a rather serious matter and must not be ignored. Unless the correct treatment is given, the delicate balance of strengths could be upset and further debilitation encouraged.

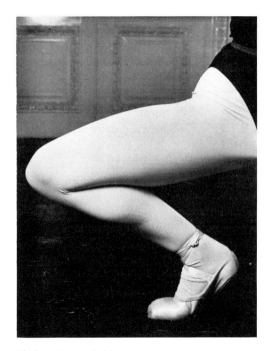

The knee in grand plié.

TORN CARTILAGE OF THE KNEE

This is usually an over-use injury, with severe pain on the inside of the joint. It is sometimes an acute traumatic injury requiring immediate medical advice. The cartilage (or meniscus) is a lining between two bones to allow them to move freely against each other. In the knee, there are two cartilages that allow the femur and tibia to glide over each other smoothly, thus absorbing most of the stresses through the knee. It is most often the cartilage on the inside of the joint that is damaged.

CAUSES

The tear tends to occur if the knee is twisted whilst it is bent. Allowing the knee to fall inwards during plié, so twisting the alignment of the leg, will either crush or tear the cartilage. The weight of the body is then incorrectly placed on the inside of the knee and not over the centre of the leg.

This injury will probably be related to poor turn-out from the hip, causing rotation in the knee joint. It may be a traumatic injury, as in landing very badly from a jump.

SYMPTOMS

Pain on weight-bearing on a bent leg; localized to the inside of the joint. There will also be some pain when rotating the lower leg outwards away from the knee whilst the knee is flexed.

The knee tends to 'lock' in a bent position, or will suddenly give way.

There may be some wasting (atrophy) of the inside thigh muscle (vastus medialis) or, in some cases, the whole quadriceps group.

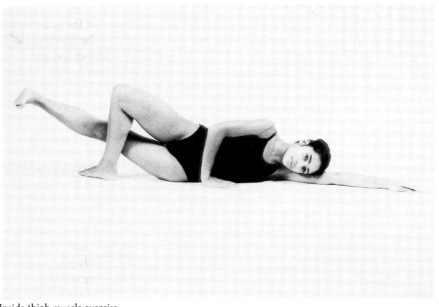

Inside thigh muscle exercise.

TREATMENT

If a lot of damage has been done and the meniscus has been badly torn, a surgeon may decide to operate.

However, if this is not necessary, physiotherapy combined with selective rest should help.

Most importantly, technique should be closely scrutinized and turn-out from the hip properly sustained.

CORRECTION

Thigh exercises to strengthen main lifting muscles, the quadriceps femoris: keeping the leg as straight as possible with the feet flexed upwards, lift the leg straight up and hold before slowly lowering and releasing.

Repetitions should be in groups of tens. As in most strengthening exercises, it is most important to do a little and often — start with two times ten repetitions and then stop and repeat at a later date. Once strength has been gained, small weights may be added on to the ankle.

Another thigh exercise: sit on a high table or chair so that the legs dangle over the edge. Slowly straighten and lift the leg with a flexed foot. Hold before relaxing and repeating.

Once the dancer is allowed to resume class work, great care must be taken not to allow the thighs to fall inwards during plié, but to keep the alignment of the leg straight.

Strength of the turn-out muscles will also help establish the correct placement of weight throughout the leg.

BURSITIS OF THE KNEE

This is an inflammation of the cushion-like pads of the knee. A bursa allows freedom of movement between a bone and a tendon and, to some extent, acts as a shock absorber.

CAUSES

Usually abuse of the kneecap, either by constant bending or by a sudden fall or blow to the knee. It can also be caused by over-use. Once a bursa becomes inflamed, it can become less spongy and degenerate.

SYMPTOMS

The dancer will complain of pain on either side of the patella. Most often on the lateral side. Pain can also be found by pressing firmly the patella, or putting direct pressure on the bursa.

There may be some swelling or local tenderness and sometimes local heat. Stairs are found to be difficult to manage, particularly when descending.

TREATMENT

Rest is often the best treatment.

Depending upon the severity of the problem, a doctor may prescribe anti-inflammatory tablets.

If the bursa has degenerated beyond help, it may be decided to remove the damaged part and so encourage the growth of new healthy tissue.

Ice-packing and ultrasound therapy from a qualified physiotherapist will also help.

Strapping may irritate the condition — if there is severe swelling, it is best not used.

CORRECTION

Once recovery is complete, a slow return to dancing is recommended, but avoiding deep knee bends and jumps. All thigh exercises should be done to maintain strength throughout recovery.

OSGOOD-SCHLATTER DISEASE

Osgood-Schlatter disease is a problem frequently found in the growing young dancer between the ages of 11 and 12.

CAUSES

It may be caused by an increase in activity and demands made upon the knees. It may occur in teenagers as they enter full-time training. The knee, to protect itself from extra pressure, will cause a bony projection to form.

SYMPTOMS

A small bump will appear, or be felt below the kneecap where ossification has occurred. Pain will be felt on most knee movements and stairs also cause pain. This condition can be detected on X-ray.

TREATMENT

Treatment is complete cessation of dancing and all weight-bearing activities.

Sometimes doctors suggest complete immobilization of the knee and even bed rest.

The amount of time needed to recover can vary between several weeks or months and it is a slow process.

CORRECTION

Once the damage has occurred, very little can be done to prevent or correct it, except for being patient! This is one instance where exercises should not be done unless a doctor advises that it is safe to begin gentle exercises.

CHONDROMALACIA PATELLAE

The name 'chondromalacia patellae' could be misleading. Similar pain is encountered in another condition called 'patella tracking syndrome'. This is when the kneecap moves incorrectly on the femur. Chondromalacia patellae is a roughening and soreness at the back of the kneecap. Usually an over-use injury.

CAUSES

In the case of patella tracking syndrome, injury is caused by a muscular imbalance so the patella is pulled too strongly off-centre. There is little apparent cause for chondromalacia patellae. The back of the kneecap becomes irritated and begins to degenerate, and may be aggravated by incorrect technique.

SYMPTOMS

Pain is felt on bending and extending the leg, and grinding may be felt.

Some slight swelling may accompany the problem.

The inside thigh muscle (vastus medialis) may appear soft and weaker than its counterparts.

The patella could feel sharp at the edges when moved gently across the knee.

TREATMENT

Rest is most important to prevent further irritation.

Doctors may prescribe anti-inflammatory tablets.

If the case is severe, a surgeon may operate to shave away the degenerated part of the patella and trim any cartilage that has become frayed.

CORRECTION

Depending on medical advice, and the actual nature of the problem, activity may irritate the knee.

If the patella is not being held properly in place, then exercises should be done as soon as inflammation has settled. Strong quadriceps exercises, such as straight leg raises should be done and increased daily. Provided the symptoms do not re-occur, gradual weight training must be encouraged to make the medial quadriceps stronger and so correct the tracking problem of the kneecap.

Dance technique must be closely re-examined to ensure that correct thigh, knee and ankle alignment is maintained.

'JUMPER'S KNEE'

A rupture or tear in the tendon that comes out of the patella and inserts into the tibia (ligamentum patellae) is referred to as 'jumper's knee'.

CAUSES

This injury tends to be found in dancers who have good elevation, hence its name, and thus tends to be found more in men than in women. The tear may be caused by dancing on a floor with a rake, so that much force is translated into the front of the knee. This may be either a traumatic or an over-use injury — frequently it is through constant excessive elevation without proper control.

SYMPTOMS

Pain is felt on jumps and knee bends.

Direct pressure onto the ligament under the patella above the tibia will locate a very tender area.

Hyperextension of the leg can also cause pain as the torn ligament tries to pull the patella flat — some swelling may also be present.

TREATMENT

Because of the nature of the injury, it may be necessary for an orthopaedic surgeon to operate and remove torn fibres or scar tissue. Recovery time, depending on medical advice, could be a few weeks. In the early stages, physiotherapy could prevent too serious an injury. Ultrasound, combined with massage across the tendon, can be very successful. Stretching and strengthening of the quadriceps will also help.

CORRECTION

Once the knee has healed and the thigh exercises have begun to strengthen the muscles, a slow and careful return to class (with very gentle jumps) can be undertaken.

In the future, the dancer must make sure that all the muscles are fully warmed up and ready for the stress of jumps in order to avoid the ligament being over-used again.

OSTEOARTHROSIS OF THE KNEE

Osteoarthrosis is a very common disease found especially in the older dancer.

CAUSES

The joint will simply begin to degenerate after many years of dancing and slowly start to wear out. It may follow repeated minor knee injuries or a cartilage removal.

SYMPTOMS

Aching, swelling and pain on most knee movements.

Arthrosis may show up on an X-ray as a narrowing of the joint space, although in the early stages, the knee may be clear on X-ray. Medical advice is essential to assess all the symptoms for a diagnosis.

TREATMENT

To some extent, the pain can be controlled by drugs and physiotherapy. With patience and sensible care, one would hope to resume some activity, even though strenuous dancing may have to cease.

CORRECTION

Some careful thinking will have to be done about how important it is to continue to dance and how much pain can be withstood. As there is very little that can be done to cure the disease, decision time has to come soon.

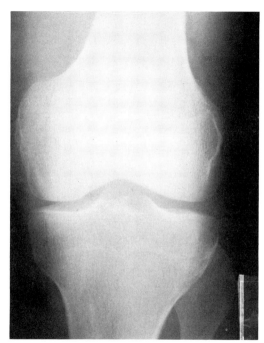

X-ray of arthritic knee joint.

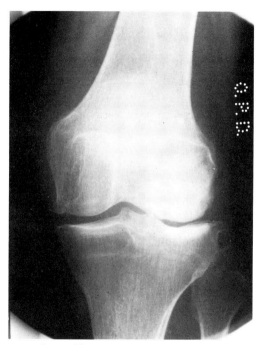

X-ray of normal knee joint.

TORN CRUCIATE LIGAMENT

This is a rather rare injury, usually traumatic with a history of either forced full extension or flexion in the knee.

There are two cruciate ligaments in the knee. The anterior (front) goes from the front of the tibia to the back of the femur, and the posterior (back) from the back of the tibia to the front of the femur. They are responsible for the stability in the knee in a forward and backward position.

CAUSES

As this tends to be a sudden injury, it may be caused by a sudden blow or fall. A collision with an object or person, with direct pressure placed suddenly on the knee, will also cause the injury.

SYMPTOMS

To see if the knee is stable, rock the lower part of the leg forwards and backwards with the dancer flat on his/her back and the leg bent at the knee to about 15° with the foot on the ground. If this is painful, or there is excessive movement, a tear or rupture may have occurred.

TREATMENT

Medical advice should be sought. Although surgery may correct and repair the damage, it is rather unlikely that the knee would stand up to dance training afterwards. The length of the cruciate ligament is most important and, if too short or too long, the leg may be unstable.

After surgery, a plaster cast may be kept

on for several weeks and rehabilitation can take up to one year.

CORRECTION

Even if surgery has been completely successful, it may be necessary to reconsider seriously the future career.

HIPS: THE HIP JOINT

The degree of turn-out in the hip joint is governed by many things. Most important of all is the angle at which the femur is set into the pelvis. The head of the femur is a round ball which is set into the socket (acetabulum) of the pelvis. Turn-out is also dependent on the elasticitiy of the 'Y' shaped ligament (the iliofemoral ligament) which holds the femoral head in place. This is the strongest ligament in the body. It has two parts: the top part runs almost horizontally, whilst the lower part is on a strong diagonal — hence its familiar name of 'Y' shaped ligament.

Turn-out is also dependent on the age at which dance training is begun. If the 'Y' shaped ligament is gently stretched at an early

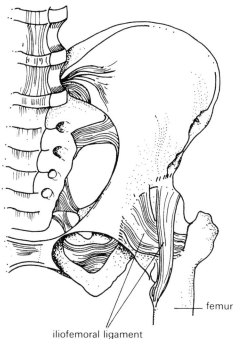

femur

iliofemoral ligament

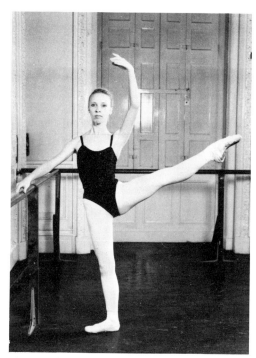

The strength of the hip socket.

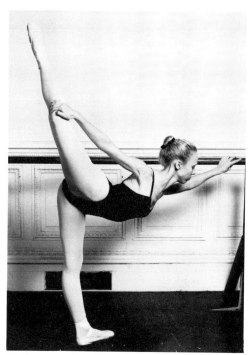

The looseness of the hip socket.

stage, it will become more elastic. The strength of the turn-out muscles round the hip will also help to maintain turn-out although the bony configuration of the pelvis will never be altered.

It is slightly easier to turn-out in the second position because the 'Y' shaped ligament is most relaxed in this position. Pliés should therefore be taught first of all in the second position.

The large muscles of the back of the hip (glutei maximus, medius and minimus) work with the strong muscles of the inner side of the thigh (adductors magnus, longus and brevis) and combine to give strength and stability to the pelvis. All these muscles work to lift the leg in a turned-out position and so it is important that they are well developed and very strong.

STRAIN OF HIP OR STRESS FRACTURE OF THE NECK OF THE FEMUR

These cause pain at the top of the leg and inside the pelvis when turning out or holding extensions to side.

CAUSES

May be caused by either poor teaching or poor technique. The neck of the femur is constantly twisted or rotated by forcing turn-out. It is possible that either one or both legs may have a stress fracture. The neck of the femur carries a tremendous load.

SYMPTOMS

Pain in the hip especially in executing movements to the side and in circular movements such as grands ronds de jambe. There may be a general aching in the hip area, or a hairline crack in the neck of the femur may appear in an X-ray, but bone scans may be required to detect a 'hot spot' to confirm diagnosis.

TREATMENT

Treatment is difficult. It is very hard to immobilize the hip and leg. The dancer should not dance until the fracture has mended according to medical advice. Very little turn-out should be used during walking or any other movements. Regular follow-up at the specialist is essential to ascertain when dancing can recommence.

CORRECTION

A stress fracture in the pelvis indicates that there may not be sufficient turn-out rotation in the hips to cope with the demand of dancing. So, unless the fracture was a freak accident, it might be wise to rethink a career as a dancer.

STRAIN OF RECTUS FEMORIS

Pain is felt in the groin at the top, front of the thigh, or anywhere along the length of the muscle to the knee.

This front and longest muscle of the four quadriceps femoris is liable either to tear or to strain.

CAUSES

Usually a traumatic injury caused by a sudden pull. It will probably have occurred when the leg was at the back and perhaps stretched too violently. It may also be an over-use injury encouraged by constant over-stretching of the leg at the back, without being properly warmed up.

SYMPTOMS

Local tenderness at the top of the thigh, with some swelling.

Pain on all leg movements to the back or even in back bends which will cause tension.

TREATMENT

Treatment is rest from class work, although some gentle floor barre work may be done. It is most important with groin injuries to allow sufficient rest time and not aggravate the problem by over-use. Some local heat may relieve symptoms. Physiotherapy may be required in the form of ultrasound and firm supportive taping in the early stages.

CORRECTION

Once symptom-free and allowed to return to class, the dancer should gently stretch the muscle to prevent this injury from re-occurring. Lie face down with the leg bent up

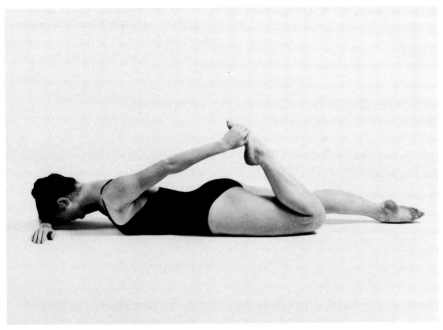

Exercise to stretch the rectus femoris.

at the knee. Holding the foot or ankle, gently pull the leg towards the body. Make very sure that there is no twist in the leg and that the thigh is parallel. This will lengthen the rectus femoris, with the dancer able to control the amount of pull. Once this becomes easier, lift the whole leg up and off the ground a few inches to increase the angle of stretch.

STRAIN OF THE ILIOPSOAS

This causes pain deep inside the groin and is often a traumatic injury caused by violent movement.

CAUSES
Like all groin muscle injuries, this is often caused by a sudden stretching when not properly warmed up. Falling into splits or over-enthusiastic leg stretching when not warmed up, could cause either a small tearing of a few fibres or a strain of the muscle.

SYMPTOMS
Pain on movements of the hip and extensions of the leg to the front.

The dancer is often unable to hold the leg in a turned-out position to the front.

TREATMENT
As this is a rather deep muscle, it is therefore very difficult to treat. Rest from any movements that cause pain or aching. Deep forms of ultrasound over the tendon insertion are useful. These must be provided by a recognized and qualified physiotherapist. Care of back posture is essential as this muscle originates in the lumbar spine and can affect the lower back.

CORRECTION
Again, it is hard to advise on corrective therapy when the muscle should be allowed to heal naturally. Gentle stretching is most important once healing has begun. Take care of the lumbar spine as strain may have started there and produced a secondary injury in the

groin. Posture is important and sitting well is also important. It is most important to realize how easy it is to strain a muscle in the groin and to warm up accordingly. Recovery can take a long time and pain-free movements tend to be rather limited.

ADDUCTOR STRAIN OF THE INSIDE OF THE GROIN

This is characterized by sudden, or maybe gradual, onset of discomfort in the fleshy part of the inside of the leg below the crotch.

CAUSES

Possibly by a change of technique — ballet to modern dance. Gradual repeated strains to the leg with poor rotation in the hip. When this is a traumatic injury it may be caused by violent acceleration or deceleration, with no previous stretching or inadequate warm-up.

SYMPTOMS

Pain on most extensions to the side, either in controlled adage movements or in grands battements.

Pain on taking off to jump, or on landing from a jump.

TREATMENT

If injury is sudden, immediate application of ice and then supportive taping by a qualified physiotherapist. Rest for about ten days. If the injury is an over-use problem, the muscular imbalance must be corrected. The thigh and turn-out muscles need to be re-educated. It is possible to work during this time provided that all painful movements are avoided.

CORRECTION

Slow, gentle warm-up when allowed to return to class. The amount of rotation in the hip should be carefully controlled and checked both with the leg straight and when bent.

HAMSTRING STRAIN

With hamstring strain, there is pain in the long muscles in the back of the thigh.

CAUSES

These muscles are responsible for bending the knee and extending the hip. An injury here is possibly caused by rapid acceleration into a jump. A sudden stretching of the leg to the front (as in grands battements) with insufficient warm up. Often occurs with a sudden loss of balance when pushing off on the leg.

SYMPTOMS

Sudden sharp pain at the back of the thigh. All extensions to the front may cause pain, possibly walking would also cause discomfort. It may manifest itself as a gradual ache following repeated minor strains to the hamstrings.

TREATMENT

In the case of a traumatic injury, immediate bed-rest for two to three days would be recommended. This would then be followed by strapping and ultrasound from a qualified physiotherapist.

CORRECTION

Gradual stretching may be done after three weeks. If the strain is a result of over-enthusiastic stretching over a long time, then it is possible to keep working with the aid of supportive taping and ultrasound treatment. Gentle stretching could then be done with the leg supported. Place the leg on a hip-level flat surface and slowly and gently pull forwards towards the leg and so stretch the hamstrings.

INFLAMMATION OF THE GLUTEAL BURSA

Pain is felt on the outside of the hip. A bursa is a protective cushion, and in this case, it works to protect the gluteus medius from rubbing against bone.

CAUSES

The bursa may become irritated and inflamed from direct impact such as a fall. It may also be caused by continual pressure from incorrect placement of the leg.

SYMPTOMS

Pain on most sideways movements and lateral rotation of the hip. Extensions to the side and circular movements (grands ronds de jambe) will also cause irritation. There may be a feeling of pressure on the outside of the hip, and local pain.

TREATMENT

Doctors may prescribe anti-inflammatory agents and perhaps recommend ultrasound treatment from a chartered physiotherapist. Some topical ointment around the hip may help relieve some discomfort.

CORRECTION

Once inflammation has subsided, technique must be closely examined and correct placement of the leg in the hip socket is most important.

OSTEOARTHROSIS OF THE HIP JOINT

This causes aching in the hip area. Generally found amongst older dancers although it may occur at any age.

CAUSES

As in most major joints in the body which are subject to wear and tear, the hip joint is likely to degenerate. A lot of extra work or damp conditions may aggravate the problem.

SYMPTOMS

Osteoarthrosis will be seen on an X-ray as a narrowing of the joint space and a degeneration of bone surfaces. Some X-rays may appear normal at first, although restriction of rotation from the hip will be noticed and so help confirm diagnosis. Pain is often felt when walking as well as when dancing.

TREATMENT

Depending on the doctor's advice, some form of painkillers may be prescribed. The degeneration of the joint will be observed by regular X-ray. It is important to keep as much mobility in the hip as possible, working with a registered physiotherapist and continuing exercises for the rest of an active life will help.

CORRECTION

Very little can be done to correct this. Rest from dancing and violent activity will help slow down the arthrosis. Mobilization of the joint as much as possible. In the end, it is up to the individual to decide how much pain and discomfort can be endured before giving up dancing.

BACK

The spine has two main functions, to act as a shock absorber and to carry the central nervous system to the brain. The spine is composed of 33 vertebrae and is divided into separate and recognizable curves.

Starting at the top, there are 7 cervical vertebrae. The first two, atlas and axis, are special as they allow the head full range of movement in all directions. The 7th cervical can be seen and felt at the base of the neck. In the thoracic curve, there are 12 vertebrae. These vertebrae also serve as attachments for the 12 ribs. There is very little forwards and backwards movement in the thoracic curve, but it does have rotation, particularly where it meets the lumbar spine. The 5 lumbar

vertebrae are slightly bigger and thicker than other vertebrae and have sideways movement, and allow movement forwards and backwards.

Below the lumbar vertebrae are 5 sacral and 4 coccygeal bones which form the posterior wall of the pelvis. These last 9 bones are fused together during early growth.

Between each vertebra are spongy, jelly-like cushions called intervertebral discs. They allow the vertebrae to move against each other and act as shock absorbers which is most important.

Any young dancer deciding to make a career in dancing must ensure that the spine has no deformities or excess curves. The teacher must look very carefully at future would-be dancers and:
  — check that the leotard or T-shirt does not have wrinkles on one side and not on the other
  — check the shape of the spine in a

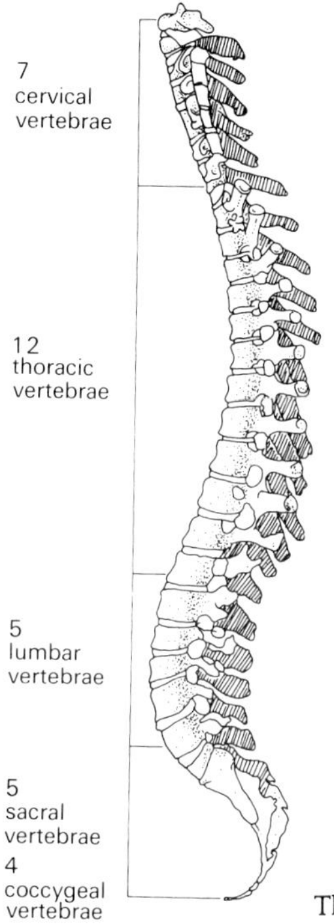

7
cervical
vertebrae

12
thoracic
vertebrae

5
lumbar
vertebrae

5
sacral
vertebrae

4
coccygeal
vertebrae

The spine.

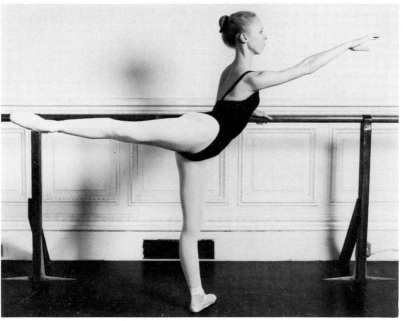

The use of the back in an arabesque.

forward relaxation in case one side of the back has an excess curve or lump of muscle.

— check the hips are at the same level and that arms fall evenly at the side.

If a girl is wearing a skirt, see that the hemline falls evenly all round.

All the above checks could help to discover a degree of spinal abnormality.

A slight degree of poor posture may be corrected by strengthening exercises but it is most unwise to attempt to train a severely abnormal spine.

If in any doubt at all about back pain, a dancer should stop all painful activities and consult a specialist. An unattended, small weakness could, eventually, lead to a major problem.

LORDOSIS

Lordosis is commonly called a 'hollow back', recognized by an excessive curve in the lumbar region.

CAUSES

Poor posture with the weight carried too far backwards. Rather weak stomach muscles would encourage the excess curve to go backwards. If the problem is skeletal, rather than postural, the child is born with this weakness in the lumbar vertebrae.

SYMPTOMS

Pain in the lower back, especially if left uncorrected until adolesence. An obvious curve in the lower back which also throws the pelvis forwards and downwards.

TREATMENT

If checked when the child is quite young and the problem is mainly caused by poor posture, corrective exercises could be prescribed. During this time, it is likely that the child would be advised not to dance until more strength is gained.

CORRECTION

Physiotherapy would encourage the back to straighten out and halt the problem. Stomach strengthening exercises may be advised to pull the body more upright and forwards. This may take several months, if not years, to correct, but a weakened spine would probably not stand up to the demands of dance training.

SCOLIOSIS

Scoliosis is a spinal abnormality causing the spine to twist sideways, often resulting in one shoulder being higher than the other.

CAUSES

A mild form of scoliosis may be caused by over-use. Always carrying a heavy bag on one side of the body or developing one set of muscles as in playing tennis or other racquet sports. A severe form of scoliosis is usually related to how the vertebrae are formed in the spine and so may be a hereditary problem or congenital abnormality.

SYMPTOMS

A visual sideways abnormality usually found in the chest (thoracic) area. The shoulders may appear to be uneven or the waistline not horizontal to the floor.

TREATMENT

Exercises designed to correct a muscle imbalance on the weakened side. It is possible that a 'brace' may be advised to correct immediately what could be a degenerative problem. Exercises and braces are of *no use* in very severe disabilities and specialist advice should be sought.

CORRECTION

Physiotherapy as medically advised. As with any spinal abnormality, correction may take a long time and it is very difficult to guarantee complete recovery.

INTERVERTEBRAL DISC LESION

Sudden pain is experienced, usually in the lower back. Popularly referred to as a 'slipped disc'.

CAUSES

The disc that separates each vertebra may be suddenly pushed out of place by a twisting movement, or a fall, or by lifting an object awkwardly. The cushion between the vertebrae then presses on the spinal cord which runs through the core of the vertebrae. The pain felt may also extend into one or both legs, as the nerves are put under pressure.

SYMPTOMS

As this is most often a sudden injury, pain tends to be rather sharp and severe. Most often found in the lumbar curve, so bends forwards or backwards may cause painful spasm, as the disc presses upon the spinal cord.

Straight leg-raising or even walking may be too painful.

Bending forwards often produces a mild curve of the back called a 'compensatory scoliosis'.

TREATMENT

Medical advice should be sought. Treatment may be total immobilization for a period of time. Traction may also be advised. If the problem is very severe, and the cartilage has degenerated, surgery may be necessary to remove the disc.

CORRECTION

As recovery is made, it is a good idea to sleep on a posture-sprung mattress. If the spine is held too rigidly in movement, and not allowed to relax into its natural curves when landing from a jump, there will be too much pressure on the lower discs. The spine must be allowed to act as a shock absorber. Remember to keep the back straight when lifting objects, and bend the knees, not the back. Do not do full sit-ups at any time afterwards.

ACHING IN CERVICAL SPINE

A general deterioration in the bones of the spine is often manifested as an ache in the neck and over the shoulder blades.

CAUSES

The most likely place for this to happen is in the 5th or 6th cervical vertebrae in the neck. It is caused by excessive and rapid head movements in pirouettes, or by over-use of head movements in general.

SYMPTOMS

Pain will be felt in the back of the neck. This may also extend to the shoulder and arm movements. The arthrosis will show up on an X-ray as a crumbling of the bone and a narrowing of the joint space.

TREATMENT

Little can be done to stop any wear and tear. Doctors may prescribe painkillers. The best advice is perhaps to stop all movements that cause pain. A collar to support the head may help, combined with mobilization (NOT manipulation of the neck) by a qualified physiotherapist.

CORRECTION

This particular injury is encouraged to develop if the dancer tends to tilt the head slightly when 'spotting' in turns. Teachers must watch carefully when dancers are first learning how to use the head movement that there is no tilting at all.

WRY NECK

Stiff necks are very common and can come on quite suddenly.

CAUSE

Usually caused by a poor sleeping posture. Upon waking, the neck is very stiff, and the head is on one side.

SYMPTOMS

Acute neck and shoulder girdle pain. There is sometimes a tingling sensation in the arm and head, or pins and needles in the area. The head is unable to turn in one direction although other movements may be possible.

TREATMENT

Physiotherapy, possibly rest in a collar to help support the head. Superficial heat to the area and gentle mobilization of cervical spine. The stiffness should have all gone in a week. No dancing should be done as it will be too painful.

CORRECTION

Careful attention to posture and sleeping position. Neck mobilization exercises should be done daily. The collar can be worn when the neck feels too tired for further work.

STRESS FRACTURE OF THE SPINE

Stress fracture is an over-use injury found frequently in the weaker lumbar curve.

CAUSES

This may be caused by constant poor posture and not allowing the spine to act as a shock absorber in jumps. Occurs more often in the male dancer because of incorrect lifting of a partner.

SYMPTOMS

Pain in the lower back, especially in jumps and lifts. There will also be pain during rest after exercise. The fracture should be visible on an X-ray but scans may be required to detect 'hot spots'.

TREATMENT

Rest from class work, but if allowed by medical opinion, a floor barre may help keep the dancer supple and strong. A body brace may be advised to keep the back immobile and take pressure off the fractured vertebra.

CORRECTION

Great care must be taken not to return to class too soon and to avoid all back bends, jumps and pointe work. As in most back injuries, stomach exercises will help strengthen the abdominal area. Sleeping on a good bed is important as it will help avoid putting too much weight on the weakened area.

SPONDYLOLYSIS/ SPONDYLOLISTHESIS

This causes low back pain and is most common in the more mature dancer.

CAUSES

This may be a hereditary complaint. It is a condition which occurs most commonly in the 4th and 5th lumbar vertebrae and is a defect in part of the structure of the vertebra. If this happens on both sides of the vertebra, the body of the vertebra may slide forwards (spondylolisthesis). Young dancers doing excessive work can produce stress in bone that leads to mild forms of backache, eventually creating this problem. Seek advice.

SYMPTOMS

As this tends to be a continuing degenerative problem, the initial pain may be no more than a general aching in the lumbar area. If the bony projection actually does slide out of place, then the pain is more severe and localized.

TREATMENT

Doctors may recommend painkillers and bed rest. This may vary from a few weeks to a few months.

Controlled work, supervised by phsyiotherapy, can help to stabilize the back up to a point, but patience is required.

In some cases, a doctor may decide to operate. By inserting a bone block or a screw between the vertebrae, the sliding forwards may be stopped.

CORRECTION

Physiotherapy would probably include stomach muscle exercises to strengthen the abdominal area. This may be a sign to cease most dance activity, or at least to decrease the workload.

RIBS

The ribs are a very important part of a dancer's body and fortunately not often injured.

There are 12 ribs attached at the back to the thoracic vertebrae. At the front the first 7 ribs are attached to the sternum. The next 3 ribs are attached to the rib above by costal cartilage. The 11th and 12th ribs are called 'floating ribs' because they are not attached at the front. Thus they tend to be more vulnerable to injury due to direct force.

CAUSE

A sudden impact into the chest wall will cause the rib cartilage to 'spring'. This may be due to a fall onto an object or a faulty pas de deux. Intercostal nerve may be damaged in the thoracic spine in the back and so cause pain.

SYMPTOMS

Sharp pain on expiration, pain on twisting movements and possibly a sensation like a bad 'stitch' in the damaged side.

TREATMENT

Rest for about 2 days until immediate pain has subsided. For sore rib cartilage it may be possible to continue work with great care not to aggravate the condition. Strong strapping during exercise will help support the area. Ultrasound from a physiotherapist will encourage recovery. In the case of intercostal nerve irritation, therapy is needed from a qualified physiotherapist to mobilize the thoracic spine. If the pain is not too severe, gentle work may be done. Recovery takes about a week.

CORRECTION

Gentle rotations of the thorax daily to restore full range of movement. Avoid lifting for about 3 weeks.

SHOULDERS —
SUPRASPINATUS TENDON

Pain is felt at roof of shoulder which is usually painful at a certain point during a movement.

CAUSE

Repeated minor injury or fall onto the shoulder. It is quite possible to have some damage to this tendon without it being too painful.

SYMPTOMS

Pain on moving arm to side against resistance. Pain when the arm is held in a horizontal position at the shoulder. Pain can be felt on pressure at the top of the shoulder.

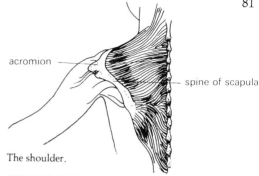

The shoulder.

TREATMENT

Ice-packs up to six times daily to reduce inflammation and ultrasound therapy with deep massage. Weight work may be done to strengthen the shoulder, once recovery from symptoms has begun.

CORRECTION

It is important that the shoulder and shoulder girdle do not weaken or become stiff, so as much mobility as possible should be encouraged.

ACROMIOCLAVICULAR JOINT

This is the joint at the roof of the shoulder between the top part of the shoulder blade and the clavicle. The 'collar bone' is held together by bands of ligaments.

CAUSE

Pain here is nearly always caused by a fall or direct blow onto the point of the shoulder.

SYMPTOMS

Acute pain in the shoulder with possible loss of arm movement and strength.

TREATMENT

If the pain is severe, removal to hospital for strapping is required. Following this, physiotherapy will help remove pain and recover movement and strength.

CORRECTION

Keep the shoulder and arm as mobile as possible without causing pain and avoid lifting and twisting movements for a while.

WARMING UP

It cannot be overstressed how important a thorough warm-up is in injury prevention. If a proper warm-up routine is done before class, the dancer will be able to move more effectively at the beginning of the class, be less likely to get hurt and be able to endure more throughout performance. Warming up increases body temperature, so that nerve impulses can travel more quickly in a warm muscle. This means that contraction and response will also be quicker. Warming up encourages an efficient rate and volume of blood circulation, which is important in the elimination of waste products from a hard-working muscle.

Any vigorous form of stretching or bouncing can result in muscle or tendon injuries and should be avoided. A slow gentle and methodical warm-up is far better. This should gently stretch main muscles in order to get them ready for fast and effective contraction, reduce any shortening of muscles that may have occurred and prepare the heart and lungs for action.

With well-trained bodies there is no real fatigue after a good 15 minute warm-up, so a dancer need not fear any resulting tiredness. In fact, a dancer would be more likely to be tired and more liable to injury if a warm-up has not been done.

Warm clothing will make the warm-up more efficient and protect from draughts and, more importantly, help keep the muscles warm once they have been worked. This is why it is important to keep warm clothing on before and after hard work, but to allow muscles to generate their own heat whilst working.

A good warm-up is imperative so far as personal freedom from injury, improved muscular co-ordination and the ability to do one's best are concerned.

COLD AND HEAT TREATMENT: SELF-HELP

Much can be done by the dancer to ease the injury and this often helps the early treatment. Immediately following an injury, whether over-use or traumatic, ice-packs should be applied. The injury should then be compressed, elevated and rested. Cryotherapy does the following:

— Decreases blood flow and therefore decreases haemorrhaging (blood in the soft tissues can be very damaging). Bruising will then be kept to a minimum.
— Decreases the metabolic activity and so decreases the need for oxygen.
— Limits the release of chemicals which causes swelling (oedema).
— Gives instant relief from pain because of its analgesic effect.

Ice should be applied for 10-15 minutes at a time, (never more than 30 minutes). If necessary, the treatment should be repeated every few hours. If there is still swelling, local fever or bruising, then the ice should be continued for the first 24-36 hours.

After the first 2 days, contrast baths may be started. A cold compress followed by a hot compress will begin to stimulate blood circulation to the injured site.

Heat treatment should be given after the first 48 hours. Heat treatment does the following:

— Increases blood circulation.
— Increases cellular metabolic activity and this aids in long-term recovery.
— Gives soothing relief and comfort.

Ice-packs may be made of crushed ice in a plastic bag. However, these should not be applied directly to the skin without the protection of some thin material, perhaps gauze or cotton. The whole injured site should then be wrapped and compressed — perhaps with a towel, and then elevated. If ice is not available, cold compresses made by running a towel under a cold water tap will do.

Heat may be applied in various forms: superficial skin sprays, hot towels or infra-red lamp. Ultrasound is another form of heat therapy which can penetrate up to 2 cm deep and must only be applied by a chartered state registered physiotherapist after consultation with a medical practitioner.

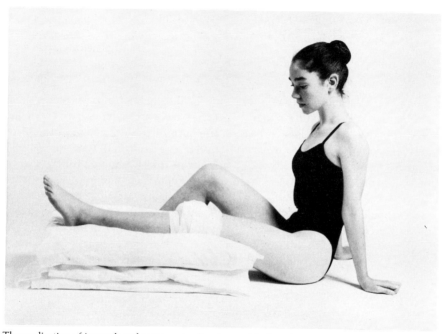

The application of ice-pack and compression bandage, with elevation.

FLOOR BARRE EXERCISES

Following an injury, it is important to follow a training routine that will maintain strength and not stress the injury. All exercises recommended for specific injuries should be done regularly during the day, gradually increasing repetition and, if appropriate, weights.

The dancer should do basic stretching and strengthening exercises on the floor to maintain suppleness and strength. Most classical exercises can be translated into floor barre exercises. As these are non-weight bearing, they can be done quite safely, provided they do not cause pain. Emphasis should be put on maintaining good posture and correct placing. These exercises can be of great value and, most importantly, the dancer can *do* something to aid recovery.

All these floor barre exercises should be done slowly and carefully, and with great emphasis on posture and placing and developing strength of turn-out. If possible, a friend or teacher should be present to ensure correct placement and to check visually for possible faults. The floor barre exercises can really help to maintain strength and flexibility and so add speed to full recovery. In fact, most of these exercises are of great value to the dancer, if done in conjunction with regular class work, and will be most beneficial in the future.

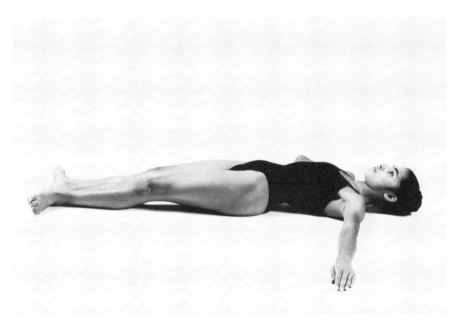

Floor barre: starting position
Feet flexed; legs turned out from the hips and the back as flat as possible. The stomach muscles should be pulled in and the arms out at the side at shoulder level.

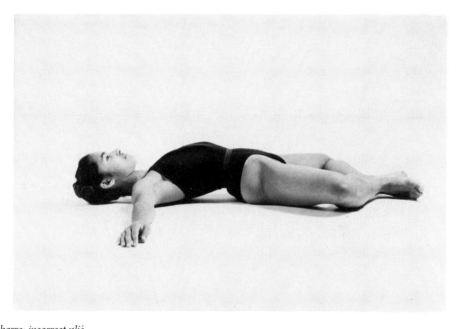

Floor barre: incorrect plié
The back is allowed to arch and the stomach muscles are not used. There is strain in the shoulders and the ankles are not supported.

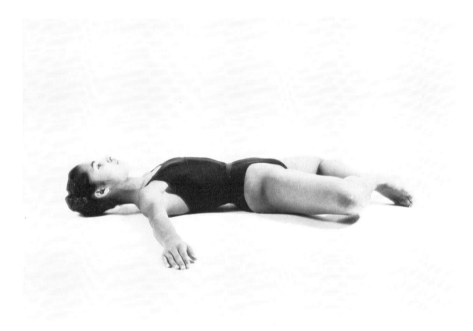

Floor barre: correct plié
Posture well maintained and turn-out controlled. Work to maintain equal turn-out of the legs, especially as they are extended. Plié should also be done in second position.

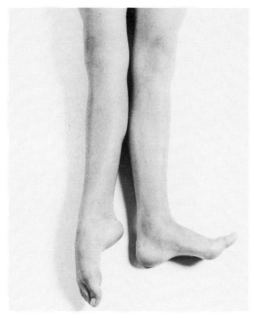

Floor barre: battements tendus
To work the foot and ankle muscles. Check for good use of the foot and guard against a sickle, however small. Repeat to the front and to the side.

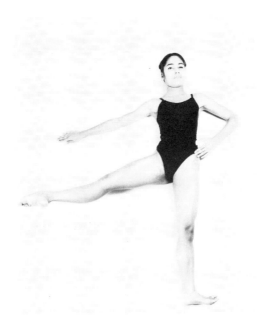

Floor barre: ronds de jambe
Slowly take the leg from the front to the side, without allowing the supporting hip to 'roll'. It may be helpful to place the hand on the hip to increase this awareness. The supporting leg should work to maintain the lateral rotation.

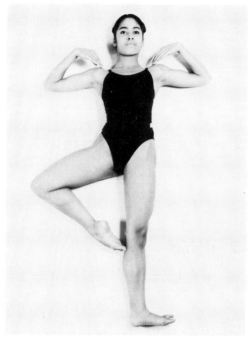

Floor barre: retiré
Draw the working leg up to retiré, checking for equal degree of turn-out at all times. Again, guard against allowing the supporting hip to move and try to keep the posture very strong. Sometimes, to discourage shoulder tension, the hands could be placed on the shoulders.

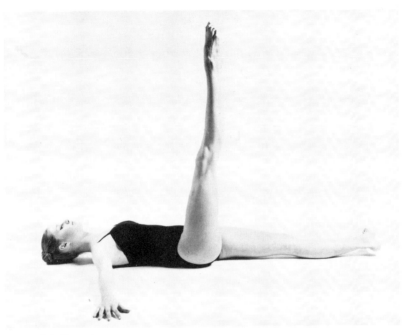

Floor barre: grands battements
Check for good posture throughout the throwing up of the leg and the lowering. The supporting side must be encouraged to keep very still and pulled up.

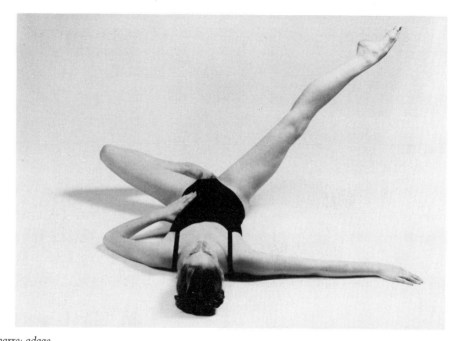

Floor barre: adage
Demi-grands ronds de jambe to improve placing and strength. As with all exercises, good posture is most important and socket rotation whilst moving the leg must be stressed. This could be practised with the supporting leg in plié to increase a sense of turn-out from the hips.

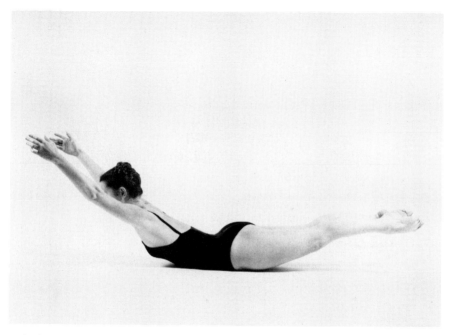

Floor barre: back exercise
To maintain strength in the back. Do not allow head and neck to strain and aim to lengthen the back. Always allow sufficient time to rest before repeating.

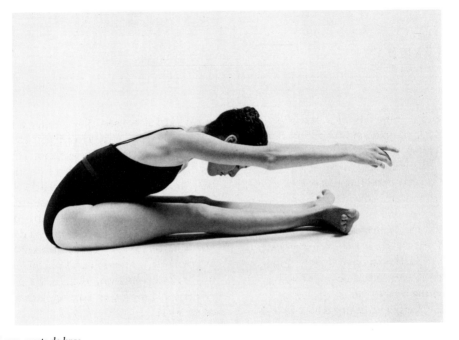

Floor barre: ports de bras
To stretch the hamstrings and spine. Try to keep the head in line with the spine and the turn-out well held in the hips.
Foot flexion will increase the degree of pull on the muscles.

CONCLUSION

Injuries will at some time be a part of a dancer's life and he or she must learn how to deal with them effectively so as to miss as little training and performing as possible. Obtaining correct and immediate treatment is of great importance and so is knowing when to stop dancing and when to be selective. An injury need not be terrible and debilitating, provided that the dancer respects the body enough to take the care and time to find out what to do to ensure recovery, and also how to prevent the injury from re-occurring. However, a long-term injury which fails to respond to all conservative treatment must seriously affect the career of the dancer and it may be necessary to have surgery. This need not be radical and, although a limb that has been operated on will not be exactly the same, an operation may resolve the problem for good and, as such, should be regarded as a welcome relief from pain. Provided dancers and teachers are fully aware of possible problems and treatment and can take responsibility for them, then the training can proceed and the joy of dancing need never be taken away.

GLOSSARY

DANCE

Adage Slow, sustained and controlled work.

Demi-Pointe A rise onto the half foot.

En Pointe A full rise onto the toes with the feet vertical.

Grands Battements A kick movement to loosen and stretch the leg.

Grands Ronds de Jambe Slow, circular movement of the leg, either from back to front or vice versa. May be done at different heights.

Plié A bend of the legs sideways with the turn out of the legs coming from the hips. May be either a half bend (demi-plié) with the heels on the floor, or a full bend (grand plié) with the heels off the floor in some of the positions.

MEDICAL

Atrophy Wasting of muscle or muscle bulk.

Bursa A cushion or sac which allows ease of movement between two surfaces.

Cartilage Connective tissue composed of various cells and fibre.

Costal Pertaining to the ribs.

Clavicle Collar bone: long, horizontal bone above first rib.

Cruciate Cross-like ligament.

Disc (or Disk) Flat, circular, jelly-like structure.

Femur Thigh bone: longest and strongest bone in the body.

Fibula Smaller outside calf bone.

Isometric Pushing or pulling against opposing pressure whilst isolating the rest of the body.

Lateral Relating to the outside or furthest side away from the centre line of the body.

Medial Relating to the inside or closest to the centre line of the body.

Metatarsal One of the 5 long bones in the foot.

Oedema (or Edema) Excessive accumulation of fluid in the tissue spaces.

Osteoarthrosis Degenerative inflammation of a joint.

Patella Flat, triangular-shaped bone, commonly called the kneecap.

Sesamoid A small, round, bony mass embedded in a tendon.

Tibia Shin bone: second largest bone in the body. The main weight-bearing bone in the calf.

Thoracic Pertaining to the chest.

Topical Treatment applied to the surface of the skin.

Vertebrae The bones of the spinal column.

BIBLIOGRAPHY

GRAY H. (1977) *Anatomy*, 15th Edition. New York, Bounty Books.

GOLANTY E. (1979) *How to Prevent and Heal Running and other Sports Injuries*. Cranbury, New Jersey; A.S. Barns. London, Tantivy.

HARRIS H. and VARNEY M. (1977) *The Treatment of Football Injuries*. London, Macdonald & Janes.

Mosby's Medical and Nursing Dictionary, 2nd Edition (1986). St. Louis, Mosby.

THOMASEN E. (1982) *Diseases and Injuries of Ballet Dancers.* Oslo, Universitetsforlaget.

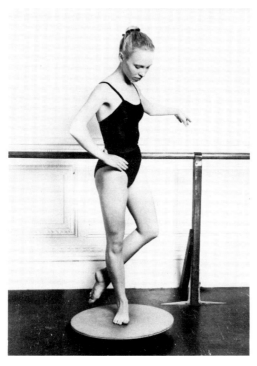

An injured dancer on the 'wobble board'.